GET INFORMED—STAY INFORMED
VACCINATIONS
Heather C. Hudak

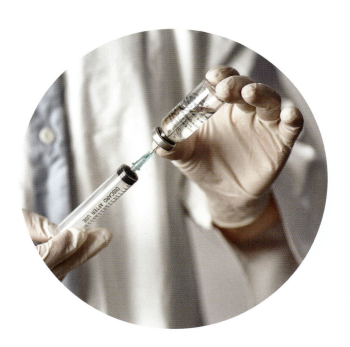

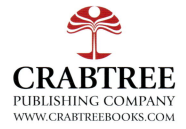

CRABTREE
PUBLISHING COMPANY
WWW.CRABTREEBOOKS.COM

Author: Heather C. Hudak
Series research and development: Reagan Miller
Editor-in-chief: Lionel Bender
Editors: Simon Adams, Ellen Rodger
Proofreaders: Laura Booth, Wendy Scavuzzo
Project coordinator: Melissa Boyce
Design and photo research: Ben White
Cover design: Katherine Berti
Production: Kim Richardson
Print coordinator: Katherine Berti
Consultant: Emily Drew, Public Librarian, B.F.A., M.S.-LIS.

Photographs and reproductions: Front cover: Shutterstock; Interior: Alamy: 11 (Chris Warham), 12 (Kathy deWitt), 39 (dpa picture alliance). Getty images: 4-5 (Robyn Beck/AFP), 13 (Dasril Roszandi/NurPhot), 19 (Alexander Ryumin/Tass), 22 (Justin Sullivan), 24-25 (Steve Pfost), 26 (Moscow Healthcare Department/Tass), 28-29 (Noel Celis/AFP), 30 (Ezra Acayan), 32-33 (Joshua Roberts), 34-35 (Arif Ali/AFP), 35 (Thierry Monasse), 36-37 Mladen Antonov/AFP), 42-43 (Saul Martinez/Bloomberg). Science Photo Library: 27 (Robert Longuehaye). Shutterstock: heading band (Rattanasak Khuentana), tablets icon (Oleksiy Mark), key and graphics tablet images, 1 (Igor Sirbu), 8-9 (Iakov Filimonov), 14-15 (Oksana Kuzmina), 18 (Rawpixel.com), 40-41 (BalanceFormCreative). Topfoto: 6 (Granger, NYC), 10 (World History Archive), 16 (Granger, NYC), 17 (Granger, NYC), 21 (ulls018566).

Diagrams: Stefan Chabluk, using the following as sources of data: p. 7 U.S. Center for Disease Control and Prevention. p. 18 Harvard Medical School/Centers for Disease Control and Prevention. p. 20 British Columbia Centre for Disease Control/RMIT University/Kylie Quinn, Damian Purcell. p. 23 Public Health Agency of Canada. p. 29 Wellcome Health Gallup World Poll 2018. p. 31 U.S. National Institute of Allergy and Infectious Disease. p. 38 World Health Organization

Produced for Crabtree Publishing Company by Bender Richardson White

Library and Archives Canada Cataloguing in Publication

Title: Vaccinations / Heather C. Hudak.
Names: Hudak, Heather C., 1975- author.
Series: Get informed--stay informed.
Description: Series statement: Get informed--stay informed | Includes bibliographical references and index.
Identifiers: Canadiana (print) 20210187743 |
 Canadiana (ebook) 20210187751 |
 ISBN 9781427150899 (hardcover) |
 ISBN 9781427150936 (softcover) |
 ISBN 9781427150974 (HTML) |
 ISBN 9781427151018 (EPUB)
Subjects: LCSH: Vaccination—Juvenile literature. | LCSH: Vaccination—Social aspects—Juvenile literature. | LCSH: Vaccination—Public opinion—Juvenile literature.
Classification: LCC RA638 .H83 2022 | DDC j614.4/7—dc23

Library of Congress Cataloging-in-Publication Data

Available at the Library of Congress

Crabtree Publishing Company
www.crabtreebooks.com   1-800-387-7650

Copyright © **2022 CRABTREE PUBLISHING COMPANY.**
All rights reserved. No part of this publication may be reproduced, stored in a retrieval system or be transmitted in any form or by any means, electronic, mechanical, photocopying, recording, or otherwise, without the prior written permission of Crabtree Publishing Company. In Canada: We acknowledge the financial support of the Government of Canada through the Canada Book Fund for our publishing activities.

Published in Canada
Crabtree Publishing
616 Welland Ave.
St. Catharines, ON
L2M 5V6

Published in the United States
Crabtree Publishing
347 Fifth Ave
Suite 1402-145
New York, NY 10016

Printed in the U.S.A./062021/CG20210401

CONTENTS

CHAPTER 1 A CONTROVERSIAL ISSUE 4
How vaccines work and how they are used; why some people choose not to use them; why not everyone has access to vaccines.

CHAPTER 2 HOW TO GET INFORMED 8
Where to find information about vaccinations; the different types of source materials; evaluating information; dealing with bias and misinformation.

CHAPTER 3 THE BIG PICTURE 14
The early history and development of vaccines and vaccinations; an understanding of antigens, antibodies, and the human immune system; herd immunity to protect whole populations; vaccination programs; side effects and outcomes of vaccines.

CHAPTER 4 MAKING AN INFORMED DECISION 24
Myths and opinions about vaccinations; different perspectives; role of health care workers, government, and nongovernmental organizations; vaccine hesitancy and anti-vaxxers.

CHAPTER 5 THE CURRENT SITUATION 36
World Health Organization's global vaccination program and initiatives; rising costs of developing and administering vaccines; problems of people not getting vaccinated.

CHAPTER 6 STAYING INFORMED 40
Guidelines and strategies for keeping up to date with new diseases and vaccines; creating your own news diet and opinions; the future of vaccine development.

GLOSSARY 44
SOURCE NOTES 46
FIND OUT MORE 47
INDEX 48

1 A CONTROVERSIAL ISSUE

Imagine you are a top athlete and you have earned a spot in an international competition. You need to visit a country where vaccinations are recommended for diseases that are not typically found in North America, such as yellow fever or typhoid. Therefore, your local vaccination program does not cover them. Why are vaccines required in some places but not others? Why are there only vaccines for certain diseases? What if you are opposed to vaccinations?

> If we imagine the action of a vaccine not just in terms of how it affects a single body but also in terms of how it affects the collective body of a community, it is fair to think of vaccination as a kind of banking of **immunity**.
>
> From the book *On Immunity: An Inoculation* by American author Eula Biss, 2015

▲ In many states, children must provide proof of vaccination, or valid reasons not to have it, before they can attend school. Free clinics in California provide vaccinations for school children who require them.

QUESTIONS TO ASK

Within this book are three types of boxes with questions to help your critical thinking about vaccinations. The icons will help you identify them.

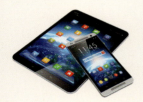

THE CENTRAL ISSUES
Learning about the main points of information.

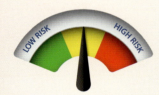

WHAT'S AT STAKE?
Helping you determine how the issue will affect you.

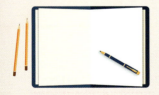

ASK YOUR OWN QUESTIONS
Prompts to address gaps in your understanding.

UNDERSTANDING VACCINES

Vaccines are substances that help protect people from diseases. They contain small amounts of the same germs that cause the diseases. Vaccines rarely make you sick, but they help you build **antibodies** and develop immunity to diseases. If you are vaccinated and still get the disease, the symptoms will likely be mild in comparison to someone who is not vaccinated.

Still, there is much debate about the use of vaccines. In North America, there are nation-wide programs to vaccinate children against certain diseases, such as polio and measles. Routine vaccines are readily available, and nearly all children take part in vaccination programs. Despite the medical benefits, some people choose not to get vaccinated for various reasons. There is increasing resistance from people who believe vaccines are harmful or that **herd immunity** is a better option. In some cases, religious or political beliefs keep people from getting vaccinated.

Many developing countries do not have the funds to provide vaccinations to everyone. People living in remote or **underserved** areas may not have good access to health services. Education programs to teach people about the benefits of vaccines may be lacking in some areas. As a result, people may fear vaccines or think them unsafe.

Before drawing any conclusions about vaccines, it is important to consider many different sources of information, facts, and viewpoints. Gaining a well-rounded understanding of the issue will help you form a balanced **perspective** or opinion.

5

VACCINE AWARENESS

Scientists continuously study and track diseases to help stop their spread and to keep people safe. One of the most effective ways to do this is through the use of vaccines. For instance, polio **outbreaks** reached a peak in the United States in the early 1950s. The disease caused paralysis in more than 15,000 people each year. After a vaccine was released in 1955, cases dropped significantly (see page 17). By 1965, there were just 61 cases of paralysis due to polio.

> "I think that the discoveries of antibiotics and vaccines have contributed to the improvement of the quality of life, making it possible to prevent **contagious** diseases."
>
> Professor Shinya Yamanaka, winner of the 2012 Nobel Prize in Physiology or Medicine, on what he believes to be the biggest life-enhancing scientific development.

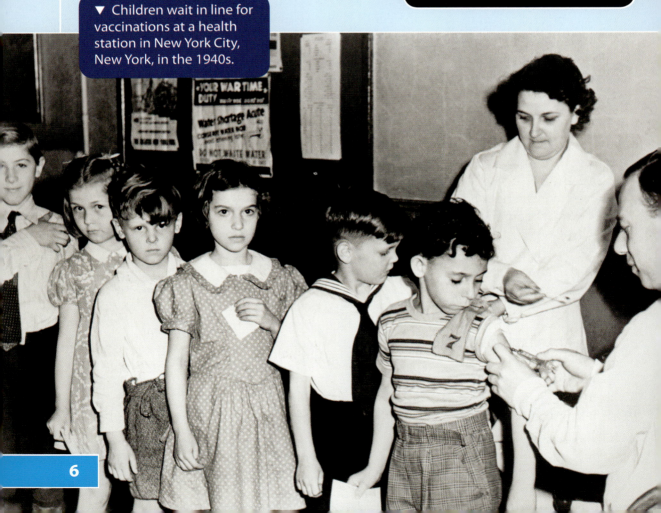

▼ Children wait in line for vaccinations at a health station in New York City, New York, in the 1940s.

According to the World Health Organization (WHO), vaccination programs prevent two to three million deaths each year. In addition, vaccines help reduce the pressure on health care systems that treat injuries and provide care for those who become sick with diseases. Vaccination programs are some of the most cost-effective public health ventures. However, they are not available in all parts of the world.

GLOBAL CHALLENGES

About one-and-a-half million children across the globe die each year from vaccine-preventable diseases. On top of that, several countries report decreases in vaccination coverage in recent years — some due to supply and storage challenges and others as a result of myths surrounding vaccine use.

People often accept poor or wrong information either out of a mistrust of science or a lack of understanding. This can create inaccuracies and **bias** in how people view topics such as vaccinations. Once you get informed about a topic, it's important to stay informed as facts, evidence, and theories about it change over time. Being informed will help you understand the world around you. It will allow you to see the impacts global events have on everyone's lives so you can make suitable decisions for humankind's future. Vaccination is currently one of the hottest topics in the news.

DISEASES PREVENTABLE BY VACCINES

Year	Disease
1798	smallpox
1885	rabies
1896	typhoid
1896	cholera
1897	plague
1923	diphtheria 🧍
1926	pertussis (whooping cough) 🧍
1927	tetanus 🧍
1927	tuberculosis
1945	influenza 🧍
1953	yellow fever
1955	poliomyelitis 🧍
1963	measles 🧍
1967	mumps 🧍
1969	rubella 🧍
1970	anthrax
1975	meningitis
1977	pneumonia 🧍
1980	adenovirus
1981	hepatitis B 🧍
1985	haemophilus influenzae type B 🧍
1992	Japanese encephalitis
1995	hepatitis A 🧍
1995	varicella 🧍
1998	Lyme disease
1998	rotavirus 🧍
2006	human papillomavirus
2019	dengue fever
2021	coronavirus

Vaccines highlighted 🧍 are part of most standard vaccination programs for children.

(Increasing length of lines only shows gradual build up of vaccine treatments available to doctors to prevent diseases.)

Vaccines developed or licensed in U.S.A.
Source: U.S. Center for Disease Control and Prevention

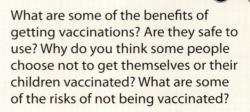

THE CENTRAL ISSUES

What are some of the benefits of getting vaccinations? Are they safe to use? Why do you think some people choose not to get themselves or their children vaccinated? What are some of the risks of not being vaccinated?

7

2 HOW TO GET INFORMED

In our interconnected, multimedia world, information is all around us. Learning about an issue such as vaccinations can be overwhelming. From TV news programs to websites and social **media**, how do you know where to look for reliable, factual details about it? The best place to start is by building up your background knowledge of the topic. It is important to find out when the issue began, who the key players are, and any important events that have already taken place.

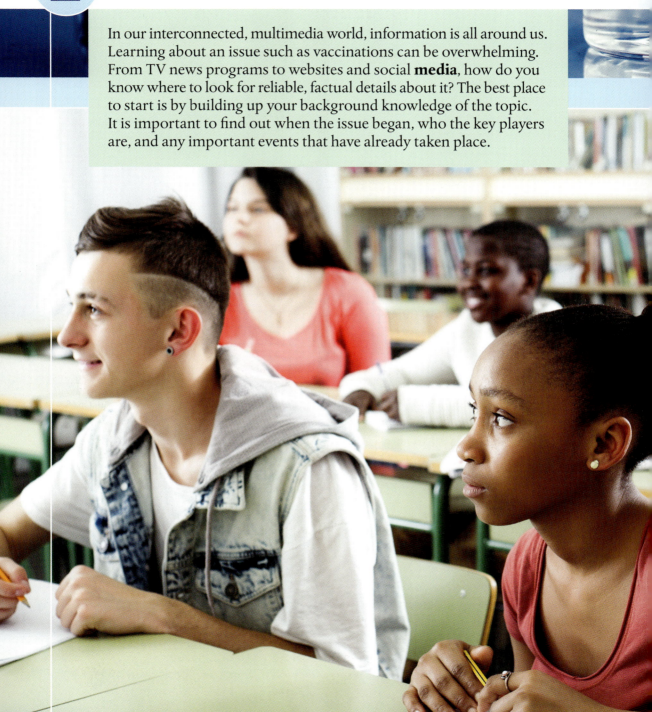

KEY INFORMATION

Vaccines are substances that stimulate the production of antibodies to help protect a person from diseases.

Vaccinations or **inoculations** are how vaccines are introduced into the body such as through injections or oral doses—those taken by mouth.

Immunization is a process in the body that happens after a vaccine is given to a person. It helps the body build immunity, or the ability to fight infections and resist diseases.

Herd immunity takes place when a major percentage of the population becomes resistant to a disease, reducing the risk of infection to people who have not been vaccinated against it or are not immune. Approximately 95 percent of a population needs to be vaccinated to stop the chain of transmission and achieve herd immunity (see pages 18, 31).

◀ Learning and sharing information in the classroom will help you shape your point of view and gain skills in **analyzing** and interpreting different types of data. A topic such as vaccinations is likely to stimulate a variety of opinions. Explore each one.

WHERE TO LOOK

Libraries are great places to find background information. They offer a wide variety of sources, including books, magazines, video recordings, newspapers, and more. Librarians are very knowledgeable about the available resources and can help you find what you need to build an overview of the current state of affairs.

Archives are another excellent resource. Many colleges and universities, museums, government agencies, and **historical societies** keep records, artifacts, and other materials in their archives. You can also find specific information about vaccinations in medical schools, where large public-health databases are held. They are organized in a way that makes it easy to search for and retrieve specific information using keywords and filters. You can also do a targeted search for information about vaccinations on the Internet using a search engine such as Google. However, keep in mind that anyone can post information on the Internet and not all of it is true.

Look for experts on the topic of vaccines, such as doctors, scientists, and local health practitioners, who share science-based research and information through social media, personal websites and blogs, or TV and radio programs. Other **credible** sources of information include **nongovernmental organizations** such as the World Health Organization (WHO); government agencies, including the Centers for Disease Control and Prevention (CDC); and university research centers, such as Johns Hopkins University.

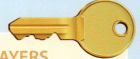

KEY PLAYERS

The **World Health Organization (WHO)** is an agency of the **United Nations (UN)**. Its purpose is to build a better, healthier future for everyone in the world. WHO works with 194 member states to create procedures, **policies**, and practices that ensure the health and safety of people everywhere.

One of the WHO's major areas of responsibility is to promote vaccination programs in parts of the world that have weak health care systems. The WHO also helps develop guidelines for vaccine development, testing, safety, and **efficacy**.

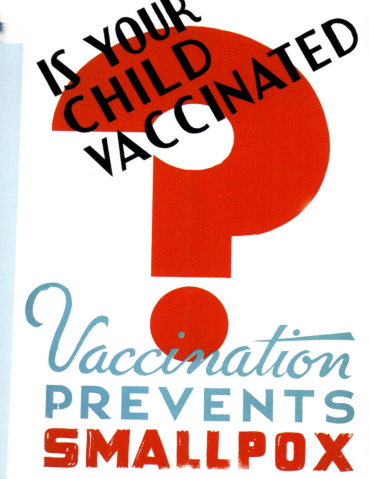

▲ Vaccination posters, such as this one from the Chicago Department of (Public) Health in 1939, can be primary sources of information.

> If you're a parent, it's not a choice whether or not you put your child in a car seat when you drive them in the car. If you own a firearm and you have children, you have to keep the firearm locked. It [should not be] a choice whether you vaccinate your children. They have a fundamental **human right** to be protected against deadly infections.
>
> Peter Hotez, Director of the Texas Children's Hospital Center for Vaccine Development at Baylor College of Medicine, 2018

SOURCES OF INFORMATION

Source materials are any items that provide knowledge about a topic. They can be a photograph, a speech, a book, or even an e-mail. You will come across countless source materials each day. They fall into three categories: primary, secondary, and tertiary.

PRIMARY SOURCES

Primary sources are original information created by people with first-hand knowledge of a person, place, event, or issue. They present eyewitness accounts or personal perspectives on the topic. Primary sources related to vaccinations include:
- travel vaccination cards from clinics
- medical journals written by doctors
- posters promoting local vaccination programs
- brochures highlighting the benefits of vaccinations
- survey results detailing the numbers of people who have been vaccinated
- news conferences with health experts and government officials
- lab results from testing new vaccines, blog posts by health care specialists, or anti-vaccination groups sharing their unique points of view online.

SECONDARY AND TERTIARY SOURCES

Secondary sources are mostly information based on primary sources. They may describe, analyze, reorganize, or **synthesize** original information in a new way. Artwork inspired by a past event, or newspaper and magazine stories written by someone who did not experience the situation themselves, are examples of secondary sources. Biographies, reference books, movies, and textbooks are other examples. Secondary sources in visual form include graphs, tables, diagrams, and charts that help make sense of complex facts, **statistics**, and processes.

Tertiary sources help guide you to primary and secondary sources where you can find more information on a topic. They include catalogs, record cards, indexes, and journal abstracts.

▲ People vaccinated for yellow fever are given an international certificate of vaccination. For health reasons, this primary source document is required for travel into some parts of the world.

EVALUATING A SOURCE

It is not enough to simply find source materials. You must ensure their credibility. Sometimes, people alter the facts to be viewed in ways that are not accurate. A few do so intentionally to try to sway others to their point of view. Others may do so out of a lack of understanding of the facts or the science involved in an issue such as vaccinations.

As a general rule, information that comes from education institutions, governments, and respected professionals is credible. However, even trusted scientists and medical experts can make mistakes or gain access to new information that changes their perspective on the issue. These are just a few of the reasons why it is important to evaluate each information source.

Follow these guidelines to determine if the source is valid:

- **Up to date**

When was the source created? Are the ideas and information outdated? Are there newer facts and figures?

ASK YOUR OWN QUESTIONS

The next time you evaluate a source of information, ask yourself if it answers these key questions to ensure it provides the complete picture: Who? What? Where? When? Why? How?

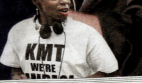

▼ In the United Kingdom, headlines in *The Guardian* newspaper grabbed readers' attention after reporting that Russian Internet trolls tried to skew public opinion in the United States on vaccine safety during the 2016 U.S. presidential election. The trolls posted fake information on social media sites.

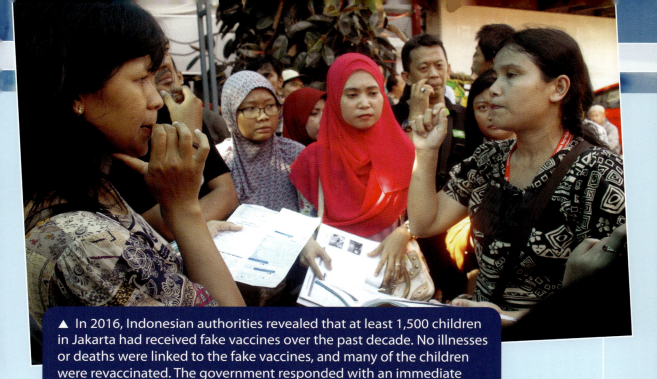

▲ In 2016, Indonesian authorities revealed that at least 1,500 children in Jakarta had received fake vaccines over the past decade. No illnesses or deaths were linked to the fake vaccines, and many of the children were revaccinated. The government responded with an immediate overhaul of the nation's food-and-drug monitoring agency.

- **Relevance**

Does the source answer your questions about vaccines and tell you what you need to know?

- **Authority**

Who created the source? Does this person have expertise about vaccines or valuable first-hand experience with vaccinations? Might they lack the qualifications of a doctor or a scientist?

- **Accuracy**

Where does the content come from? Does the author cite fact-based evidence? Can you find other sources that back it up?

- **Purpose**

Why was the source created? Was it intended to sway the reader? Does it present a strong point of view or opinion?

WATCH FOR BIAS

Bias happens when someone has a prejudice, preference, or slant in favor of or against something. It makes their arguments unbalanced. Often, these feelings are based on myths, misinformation, or **stereotypes**. Some people intentionally embed their opinions or beliefs into the information sources they create. However, in many cases, people may not even realize they are being biased toward a certain person, place, idea, or object.

If a source has a strong purpose, it may well be biased. Source creators might use a certain tone or specific words and phrases to bring out certain emotions. They may leave out some facts or details to present a limited view of the topic and create an impression.

3 THE BIG PICTURE

Illness and disease have been parts of the human experience since the beginning of time. Scientists work hard to monitor diseases and track where and when they may spread. It is important to know if there is a spike in the **prevalence** of a disease in a certain area, as it could lead to an outbreak, **epidemic**, or worse, a **pandemic**.

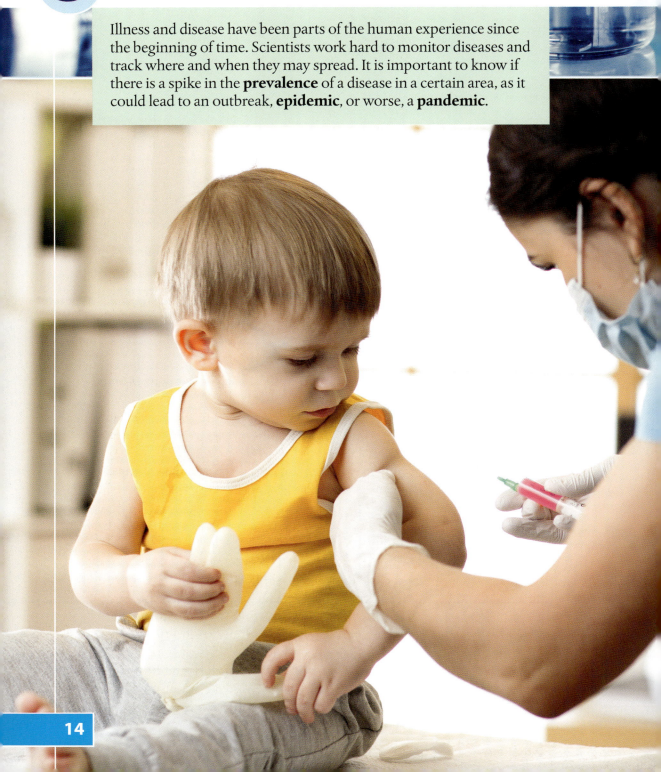

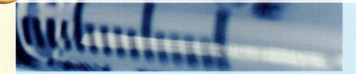

KEY INFORMATION

Infectious diseases are disorders caused by microorganisms such as bacteria, viruses, fungi, or parasites. An infection happens when microorganisms invade the body.

Epidemiology is the scientific study of the occurrence of diseases within a specific population.

When a disease is **endemic**, scientists expect to see a certain number of cases over a specific timeframe in a particular area. When there are suddenly more cases than expected, or a disease appears in an area where it doesn't normally exist, it is an **outbreak**.

An **epidemic** is the rapid spread of a disease over a large area to many people at the same time, while a **pandemic** refers to an epidemic that happens worldwide and affects a large number of people.

◄ In the United States, children can be vaccinated for as many as 14 diseases by the time they are two years old.

VACCINE COVERAGE

Prevention is important to keep people safe from deadly diseases, and vaccination is considered the most effective way to fight diseases. In fact, there are no known cures or ways to treat many vaccine-preventable diseases. They can cause serious illness, long-term disability, and even death. There are vaccines for more than 20 life-threatening diseases, and about 80 percent of children are vaccinated against common diseases in their part of the world. An increase in vaccine coverage in recent decades has led to a decline in illness and disease overall. However, millions of children around the world are not vaccinated.

OBSTACLES TO VACCINATIONS

In some countries, the health care system cannot support a vaccination program. Social barriers, such as language, culture, or location, may prevent a program from reaching people. Some religions believe disease is an act of their god or **supreme being**, and followers choose not to go against this.

Other people lack knowledge about the science behind vaccines. They have concerns over the safety of putting a foreign substance into their bodies or believe that vaccines are not as effective as getting the disease. Distrust of the government or health or aid organization that promotes or **administers** the vaccine, and misinformation spread by sources that lack credibility, are other factors. To understand the big picture of vaccination, you need to understand how vaccines work, why they are needed, and how to get them.

15

EARLY RESEARCH

Modern vaccine development began in 1796 when British doctor Edward Jenner used the cowpox virus to protect people against smallpox. Smallpox is a deadly disease that had **maimed** and killed people for thousands of years. Jenner improved on an ancient idea of inoculation, or using a small amount of a related but less harmful **pathogen** to build immunity to smallpox. It worked.

In 1853, the United Kingdom made it mandatory for babies to receive the smallpox vaccine. A parent could be fined or imprisoned for **noncompliance**. As smallpox was defeated in the Western world, health organizations set goals to wipe it out globally. On May 8, 1980, the WHO declared the world smallpox-free. Jenner is sometimes called the father of immunology for his pioneering work.

RABIES AND POLIO VACCINES

In 1881, French **microbiologist** Louis Pasteur made another leap forward when he injected an **attenuated**, or weakened, **strain** of the anthrax virus into sheep.

▼ This 1802 British cartoon is an early example of anti-vaccine views. It shows people experiencing strange side effects such as growing cattle horns, after receiving a smallpox vaccine made from the cowpox virus. However, these side effects are not known to have happened.

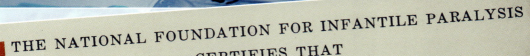

▲ Children who took part in Jonas Salk's 1954 polio vaccine trials received this certificate and pin.

After being injected with anthrax, the vaccinated sheep survived while sheep that had not received the vaccine died, proving the power of the vaccine. Pasteur also created other vaccines, including one for rabies.

The polio vaccine is one of the most notable to date. It was developed in the United States by Dr. Jonas Salk in the early 1950s. In the two years leading up to the mass use of the vaccine in 1955, there were about 45,000 new cases of polio each year in the United States. By 1962, there were just 910 new cases. But Salk's vaccine provided protection only against a certain strain of polio virus. In 1963, Dr. Albert Sabin developed a vaccine that killed all strains of the virus. It soon became the vaccine of choice for eradicating the disease around the world. Since 1988, global cases of polio have dropped by 99 percent.

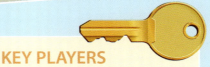

KEY PLAYERS

In April 1955, American company **Cutter Laboratories** gave about 200,000 people in the Western and Midwestern United States a defective polio vaccine it had produced. As a result, more than 40,000 people contracted polio. About 200 children were paralyzed and 10 died.

The Cutter incident raised major concerns about the safety of vaccines. It also led to anti-vaccination movements that continue to this day. In response, the U.S. government raised the standards for manufacturing and testing vaccines, and set up the National Vaccine Injury Compensation Program.

HOW VACCINES WORK

The human body is constantly under attack from pathogens found in the environment that can invade and make a person sick. The immune system helps keep people healthy. It consists of many cells, tissues, organs, and proteins that work together to protect the body from invaders. People cannot survive without a healthy immune system.

ANTIGEN AND ANTIBODIES

Each type of pathogen has a unique set of **antigens** on its surface. These molecules are a warning sign that lets the body know it is under attack. When antigens enter the bloodstream, the immune system goes into defense mode. It builds antibodies to fight against the disease by destroying or blocking the antigens.

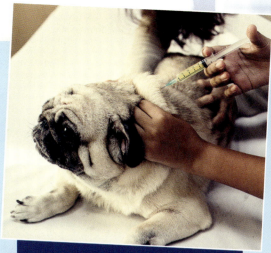

▲ Vaccinations are not only for humans. Dogs, cats, horses, cows, and other animals are also vaccinated against potentially serious and even fatal diseases such as rabies.

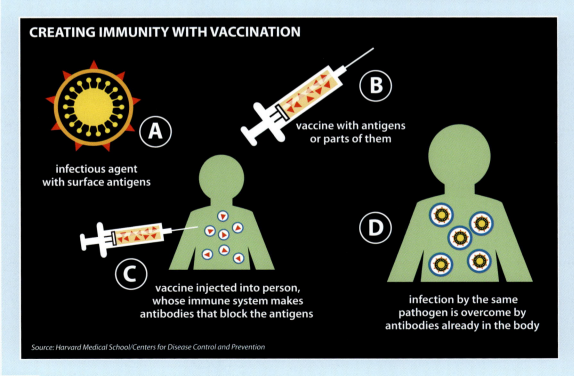

CREATING IMMUNITY WITH VACCINATION

A — infectious agent with surface antigens

B — vaccine with antigens or parts of them

C — vaccine injected into person, whose immune system makes antibodies that block the antigens

D — infection by the same pathogen is overcome by antibodies already in the body

Source: Harvard Medical School/Centers for Disease Control and Prevention

The immune system remembers every pathogen it encounters so it can fight them off stronger and faster if they enter the body again. It keeps a supply of antibodies in reserve. Vaccines mimic, or copy, the process of an antigen entering the body and stimulating the immune response.

DIFFERENT FROM DRUGS

The resulting immunization does not work the same way as drugs and other medical treatments. Instead of relieving symptoms or killing pathogens, it helps the body build a natural reaction to viruses, bacteria, and other harmful toxins, or poisons, that enter the system. Vaccines contain only a small amount of an antigen—just enough to trick the body into believing it has been infected with a disease so that it develops antibodies to fight against it. Vaccines almost always do this without making the body sick.

KEY PLAYERS

Maurice Ralph Hilleman is said to be the father of modern vaccines. He developed more than 40 vaccines while working at the Merck Institute of Therapeutic Research in West Point, Pennsylvania. He is responsible for making 8 of the 14 vaccines routinely given to children today, including the measles, mumps, and rubella (MMR) vaccine. Hilleman also served as an advisor to the WHO. He was awarded the National Medal of Science in 1988.

▼ Some vaccines are made by injecting the virus into fertilized chicken eggs then letting the eggs, incubate for several days while the virus replicates. The virus-containing fluid is then harvested from the eggs and used to make a vaccine. The vaccine may need to be stored and transported at a very low temperature to remain effective.

A LONG, EXPENSIVE PROCESS

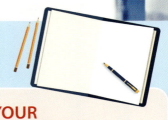

Developing a new vaccine can take many years and cost millions of dollars. There are four main types of vaccines. Live, or attenuated, vaccines contain a weakened strain of the pathogen. A person needs just one or two doses to become immune for life. Inactivated vaccines contain a killed version of the pathogen. A person may require several doses of killed vaccines throughout their lifetime. Toxoid vaccines consist of toxins the pathogen produces, while subunit vaccines are made from parts, or subunits, of the pathogen. Scientists are also working on developing **synthetic** vaccines that contain no **genetic material**.

ASK YOUR OWN QUESTIONS

Why do you think vaccines need to go through so many trials? Who pays for these trials? Why is it important for government agencies to oversee the development process? Once approved, why is it necessary to continue monitoring vaccine use and development?

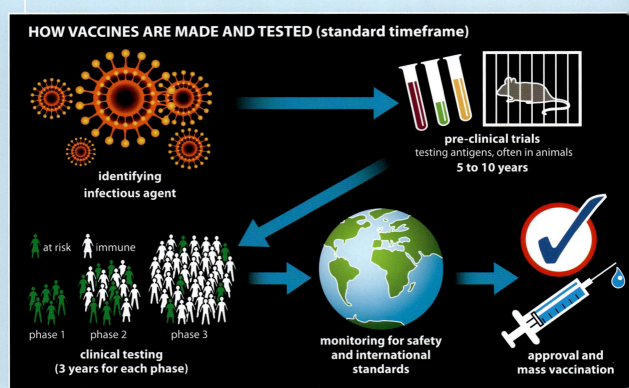

HOW VACCINES ARE MADE AND TESTED (standard timeframe)

identifying infectious agent

pre-clinical trials
testing antigens, often in animals
5 to 10 years

at risk / immune
phase 1 phase 2 phase 3
clinical testing
(3 years for each phase)

monitoring for safety and international standards

approval and mass vaccination

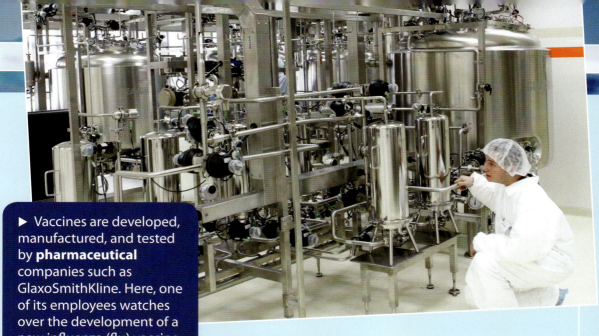

▶ Vaccines are developed, manufactured, and tested by **pharmaceutical** companies such as GlaxoSmithKline. Here, one of its employees watches over the development of a new influenza (flu) vaccine. Every effort is made to make sure the process is not contaminated by germs in the air.

VACCINE TRIALS

Once scientists have developed a vaccine, they need to perform rigorous, or extremely thorough, trials with it to ensure its safety and efficacy before it is approved for use on the general public. There are typically four trial phases. The first phase involves inoculating about 100 healthy people who are not likely to experience any complications from the vaccine. If successful, phase two involves vaccinating hundreds of members of the target population. If the vaccine achieves immunity safely, scientists begin phase three trials.

APPROVAL PROCESS

Many thousands of people from various social and ethnic groups and locations are given the vaccine to ensure it will work equally well on a mix of people in a range of environments. In the United States, success at phase three leads to approval from the Food and Drug Administration. But the vaccine must still go through another approval by vaccine experts who advise the Centers for Disease Control and Prevention (CDC) on its ability to work before it can be made publicly available. Other countries including Canada have a similar system.

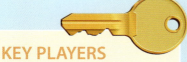

KEY PLAYERS

The U.S. Food and Drug Administration (FDA) is responsible for ensuring the quality, safety, security, and efficacy of any medical devices and treatments, including drugs and vaccines. Within the FDA, the Center for Biologics Evaluation and Research (CBER) **regulates** vaccine products under federal law. It promotes the safe use of vaccines and provides information to the public for this purpose.

VACCINATION PROGRAMS

Each country has its own vaccination program, schedule, and recommendations. The local health authority issues guidelines as to which vaccines are offered generally or are available on request, and when. The vaccines a person receives depends on a number of factors, including age, lifestyle, health conditions, location, job, and whether they have received previous vaccinations.

In the United States, people have access to vaccines for 17 diseases, including rubella, tetanus, hepatitis A and B, and whooping cough (pertussis). Most are administered in the first 15 months of a person's life since a child's immune system is not yet fully developed and children are at the highest risk of getting sick from diseases.

THE CENTRAL ISSUES

Imagine you were born in another country and later moved to North America. You missed some of your recommended vaccinations as a child as a result. What would you do? Would you get your vaccinations later in life? Would you wait to see if there was an outbreak of the related disease first? Why does it matter?

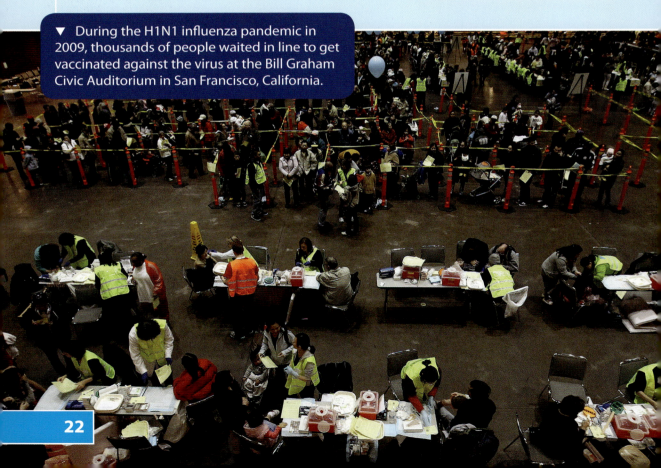

▼ During the H1N1 influenza pandemic in 2009, thousands of people waited in line to get vaccinated against the virus at the Bill Graham Civic Auditorium in San Francisco, California.

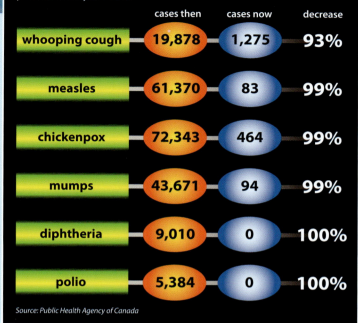

> *The return on investment in global health is tremendous, and the biggest bang for the buck comes from vaccines. Vaccines are among the most successful and cost-effective health investments in history.*
>
> Seth Berkley, CEO of Gavi, in a *Huffington Post* article in December 2011

AGE- AND TRAVEL-RELATED

Teens and adults may need to receive **boosters**, or additional doses of vaccines, throughout their lives to ensure their immunity. In addition, some vaccines are designed specifically for diseases that target teens or adults. Others, such as the flu vaccine, are given annually since the strain of the virus targeted by the vaccine changes often. Most vaccines are administered via injection. Some are given orally or are sprayed into the nose or mouth.

Certain diseases may not occur or be a widespread threat in some countries. For instance, yellow fever is rare in Canada or the United States, so people living in these countries do not typically receive this vaccination. If they travel to another part of the world where yellow fever occurs, they may be required to get the vaccine to help prevent the spread in that country and reduce the risk of bringing the disease back with them.

SAFETY AND SIDE EFFECTS

Vaccines are safe to use but can cause side effects in some cases. Most of the effects are minor and go away on their own after a few days. They vary from one vaccine to another and include fatigue, swelling, or redness at the injection site, hives, or headache. Typically, the risk of not getting a vaccine for a disease is much greater than the risk of any side effects. For example, about one in a million doses of the MMR vaccine lead to a bad **allergic reaction** compared to 139 motor vehicle deaths per one million people.

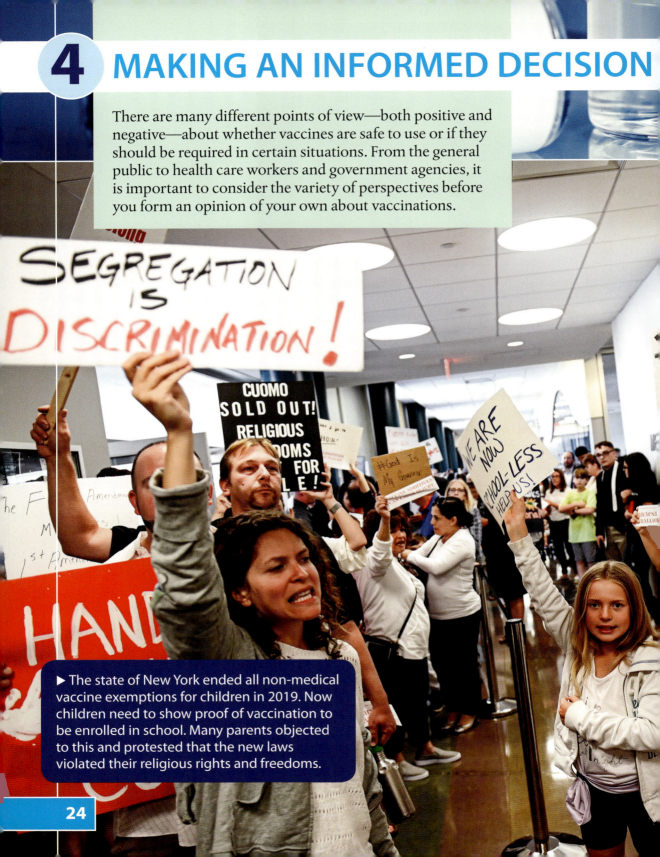

4 MAKING AN INFORMED DECISION

There are many different points of view—both positive and negative—about whether vaccines are safe to use or if they should be required in certain situations. From the general public to health care workers and government agencies, it is important to consider the variety of perspectives before you form an opinion of your own about vaccinations.

▶ The state of New York ended all non-medical vaccine exemptions for children in 2019. Now children need to show proof of vaccination to be enrolled in school. Many parents objected to this and protested that the new laws violated their religious rights and freedoms.

WHAT'S AT STAKE?

There is scientific evidence that shows vaccines save millions of lives each year and pose minimal risks. People who are not vaccinated put themselves and others at risk. Knowing this, should people be given the choice to opt out of vaccinations? Should they be required to get them even if they are opposed to them or it goes against their beliefs?

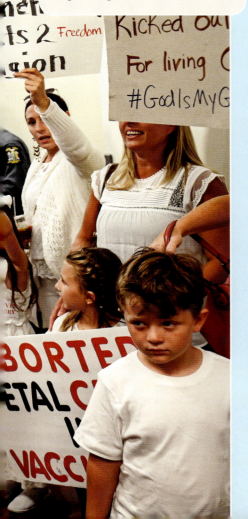

ASSESSING INFORMATION

To be a lifelong learner and make informed decisions, you must know how to evaluate information critically and competently. Anyone can post a blog online, independently publish a book, or create a brochure to hand out in the streets. The information may not be accurate or high quality. You need to know how to analyze and interpret the source to ensure its validity and credibility. For this reason, developing information literacy skills is important when learning about vaccinations and other **current events**.

MYTHS AND OPINIONS

First, you must distinguish facts from myths or opinions that are based on a person's feelings and cannot be proven right or wrong. An example of a myth would be to say that most diseases children are vaccinated against are not serious. Yet there is clear evidence that all diseases children are vaccinated against can cause serious illness or even death. Facts show that for every 1,000 people who contract measles, one or two will die. So draw conclusions only after thorough investigation.

Information literacy includes making a list of any questions you have and looking for appropriate source materials to answer them. Gather a range of information from reliable sources, sort them, select the key items, and use your time wisely and effectively to draw up an opinion, a view, or conclusion as needed. Constantly review your position as new information comes to light. As new facts arise, opinions may change.

TO VACCINATE OR NOT

Many factors contribute to whether a person is vaccinated or not. Parents and guardians are legally responsible for the health and well-being of their children. Where available, most choose to take part voluntarily in vaccination programs as prescribed by local health care systems. Based on scientific evidence, they believe vaccines are the best way to protect their children from becoming seriously ill or dying. Without vaccines, even diseases that are rare or seemingly harmless, such as tetanus, are potentially deadly.

PROTECTING OTHERS
In addition to keeping children safe, vaccinations help prevent the spreading of infectious diseases. Certain diseases can spread rapidly through the air, food, water, **feces**, or contact with infected animals.

ASK YOUR OWN QUESTIONS
During the COVID-19 pandemic in 2020, how did the global **economy** suffer? Why did businesses need to close and many people stop working? What impact did it have on health care and education? How could a vaccine have helped?

▼ Passengers at the main airport in Moscow, Russia, were subjected to heightened health-and-safety measures due to the COVID-19 pandemic in 2020. Without a vaccine, extra precautions were put in place to help prevent the spread of the deadly virus.

▶ Government health department and pharmaceutical company posters are sometimes used to raise awareness about vaccination programs and their benefits.

Even one case of a highly contagious disease, such as COVID-19 or Ebola virus, can lead to an outbreak. When people delay or refuse to get a vaccine, they put others at risk, especially those with weakened immune systems and other **chronic** medical conditions. Newborns and the elderly are also more vulnerable and are less able to fight off complications due to vaccine-preventable diseases.

WHAT TO BELIEVE?

In recent years, an increasing number of **sensationalist** news stories and social media posts have caused some people to question whether they should have their children vaccinated. These stories often contain personal opinions or false information. Reading about fake vaccines in Indonesia (see page 13) or hearing a podcast about a historic event, such as the Cutter incident (see page 17), can have a major effect on the decision-making process.

Despite the facts about vaccine safety and efficacy, parents and guardians may find it difficult to make an informed decision as a result. Another reason some people choose not to participate in vaccination programs is because they think vaccines cause more harm than good, and the risks of side effects outweigh the benefits.

VACCINATION HESITANCY

A growing number of people are choosing not to vaccinate their children or get vaccinated themselves, or to delay vaccination even when it is offered or is readily available. Vaccine hesitancy, also known as anti-vaccination or anti-vax, is often supported by organizations that have an interest in discrediting vaccines. They may even pay for ads to help spread their message.

Religion is one of the top reasons for anti-vaccination. Even though people may be well educated about the benefits of vaccines and even agree with them, they may still choose not to get vaccinated because it conflicts with their religion. In most states, religion is an acceptable reason not to get vaccinated even if it is mandatory.

PERSONAL BELIEFS

Some people think contracting a disease provides better immunity than vaccination. Others believe that the vaccine will not work anyway. A third group thinks there is no need to vaccinate against rare diseases since the likelihood of contracting them is so low. A few believe the risk of serious illness is unlikely or that modern medicine will be able to treat them successfully if they fall ill. They may even think maintaining a healthy lifestyle will keep them safe. Most health authorities do not consider these valid reasons for anti-vaccination.

LACK OF TRUST

There are yet other people who believe vaccines are a money-making scheme for pharmaceutical companies. This notion has some legitimacy due to the industry's reputation for charging high prices, replacing older drugs with newer ones that cost more, faking data, and more. These issues create a lack of trust among the general public.

KEY PLAYERS

In 1998, **Dr. Andrew Wakefield**, a British surgeon and medical researcher, published a case study that falsely claimed the measles, mumps, and rubella (MMR) vaccine was linked to autism.

The case study received a great deal of attention. As a result, many parents chose not to vaccinate their children, and measles cases increased across the United Kingdom, Europe, and North America. Soon after, more studies were published showing Wakefield's claims were scientifically incorrect. Later, it was shown that Wakefield's research had been funded by lawyers who were representing a group of anti-vaxxers.

Wakefield was found guilty of several charges and lost the right to practice medicine in the United Kingdom.

▶ During 2016 and 2017, about 800,000 children in the Philippines received a new vaccine for dengue fever, a viral disease. The vaccine may have been harmful to anyone who had not already been infected with the virus. It put them at greater risk than if they had not been vaccinated at all. Some families, pictured here, blamed the vaccine for their children's deaths.

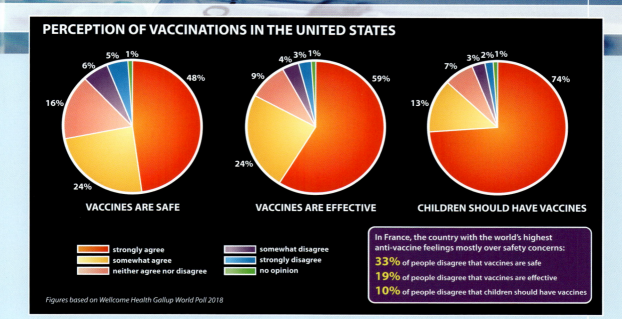

PERCEPTION OF VACCINATIONS IN THE UNITED STATES

VACCINES ARE SAFE: 48% strongly agree, 24% somewhat agree, 16% neither agree nor disagree, 6% somewhat disagree, 5% strongly disagree, 1% no opinion

VACCINES ARE EFFECTIVE: 59% strongly agree, 24% somewhat agree, 9% neither agree nor disagree, 4% somewhat disagree, 3% strongly disagree, 1% no opinion

CHILDREN SHOULD HAVE VACCINES: 74% strongly agree, 13% somewhat agree, 7% neither agree nor disagree, 3% somewhat disagree, 2% strongly disagree, 1% no opinion

Legend: strongly agree, somewhat agree, neither agree nor disagree, somewhat disagree, strongly disagree, no opinion

In France, the country with the world's highest anti-vaccine feelings mostly over safety concerns:
33% of people disagree that vaccines are safe
19% of people disagree that vaccines are effective
10% of people disagree that children should have vaccines

Figures based on Wellcome Health Gallup World Poll 2018

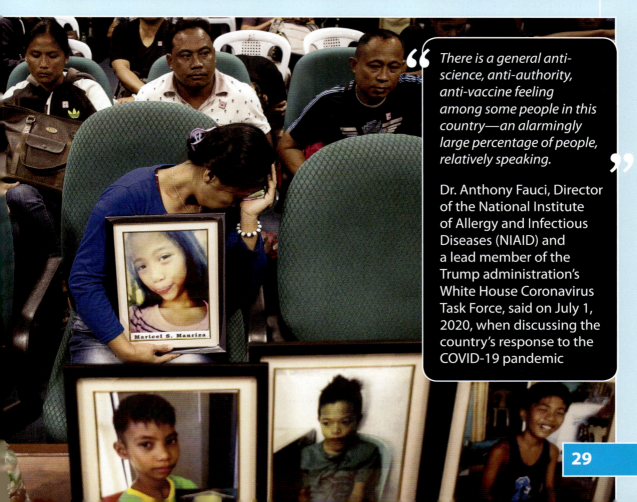

"There is a general anti-science, anti-authority, anti-vaccine feeling among some people in this country—an alarmingly large percentage of people, relatively speaking."

Dr. Anthony Fauci, Director of the National Institute of Allergy and Infectious Diseases (NIAID) and a lead member of the Trump administration's White House Coronavirus Task Force, said on July 1, 2020, when discussing the country's response to the COVID-19 pandemic

THE ROLE OF HEALTH CARE WORKERS

As vaccine hesitancy becomes more common, it falls to physicians, pharmacists, and other primary health care providers to raise public awareness of vaccination programs and to inform people about the safety, efficacy, and benefits of vaccines. One of the key ways they do this is by providing scientific evidence that dispels myths in a way that is respectful and without judgment.

To do this effectively, health care professionals must be well informed themselves and also have confidence in vaccinations, which is not always the case. In some instances, they feel unprepared to answer questions and address concerns.

ASK YOUR OWN QUESTIONS

What are the advantages and disadvantages to herd immunity? What role do vaccines play in herd immunity? What can health care workers do to better educate people about herd immunity through a vaccine?

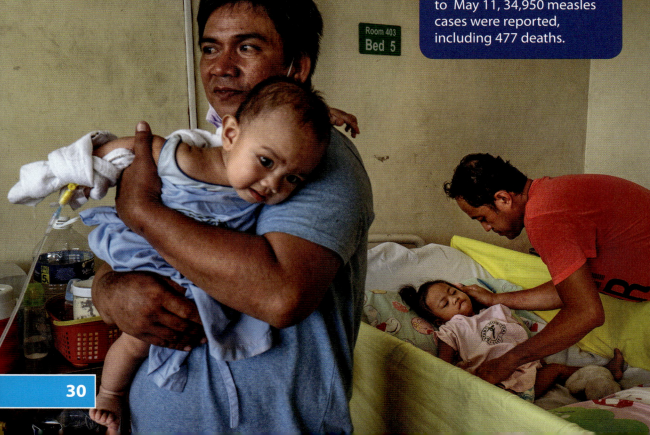

▼ The Department of Health in the Philippines declared a measles outbreak in 2019. From January 1 to May 11, 34,950 measles cases were reported, including 477 deaths.

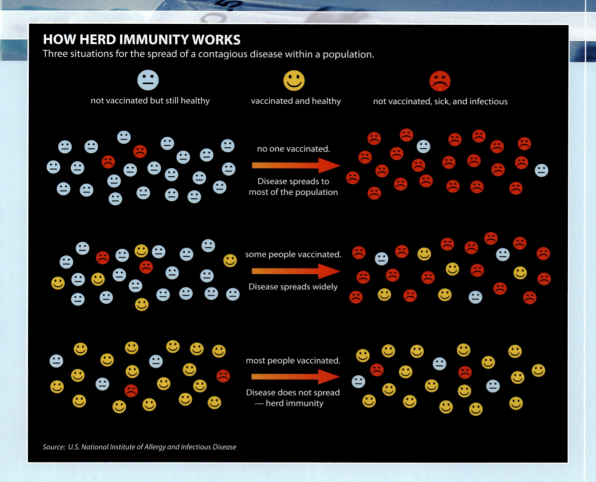

Source: U.S. National Institute of Allergy and Infectious Disease

Typically, vaccinated health care workers, people who have had positive vaccine experiences, and people who have more knowledge about vaccines, are more likely to recommend vaccines.

SUPPORTING THE CAUSE

The majority of American and Canadian doctors believe vaccines are some of the safest forms of medicine available. There is a medical consensus that herd immunity via vaccination is the best way to protect communities against diseases.

Most medical professionals also agree with current vaccination standards and would vaccinate their own children according to them. Some physicians have gone so far as to ban patients who do not agree to take part in the recommended vaccination programs.

Others, though, believe their patients should have the freedom to choose for themselves whether to be vaccinated. There are also doctors who believe children get more vaccines than they need. There is also a very low percentage of medical professionals who are anti-vax.

GOVERNMENT GAINS

Governments often invest in vaccine development for the greater good of society. Vaccines can ease pressure on health care systems by reducing illness and boosting economic stability. It takes a large amount of time and money to care for the sick. Vaccines to prevent people from becoming ill in the first place are a much more affordable option. For example, the polio vaccine, costs as little as $1 per dose, whereas treatment for a person who contracts polio can cost thousands of dollars.

WHAT'S AT STAKE?

Some people argue government-required vaccinations go against an individual's rights and freedoms. Others suggest it keeps each person from making decisions that put themselves and their families at risk, much like the required use of car seats or seat belts. Should parents have the right to opt out of vaccination programs for their children? Should they face penalties if they do? What are the risks?

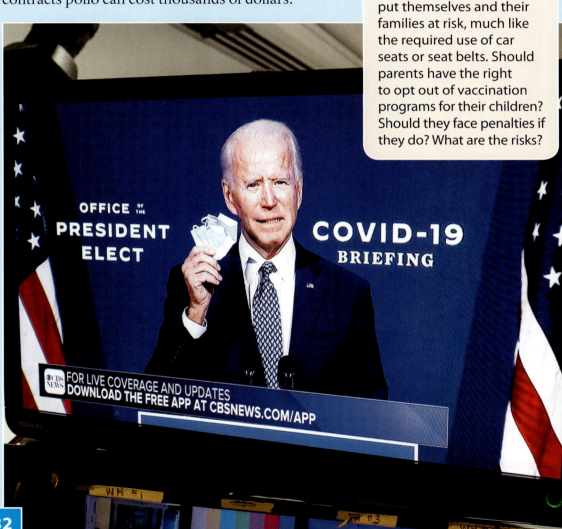

HEALTH CARE OVERLOAD

When many people become sick with the same disease all at once, local hospitals and clinics can become overrun with patients. There may not be enough resources and health care workers to care for everyone. On top of that, people who become seriously ill may not be able to work and actively contribute to the economy. School attendance may decline. There may be a large financial loss for individuals and organizations when people take time off from work due to sickness or to care for a family member. In a pandemic where no vaccine exists, such as COVID-19 in 2020, governments are forced to shut down schools and most businesses to protect as many people as possible. This has disastrous effects on the economy and well-being of populations.

As a general rule, when health improves, economies grow. Healthy children perform better at school, and healthy adults are more productive at work. As such, vaccines are considered an important and often essential preventive health care measure.

EDUCATION AND ADMINISTRATION

Often, governments can be relied on to provide factual information to help educate people about the benefits of vaccines. They play a key role in implementing vaccination programs and regulating vaccination production and use to ensure vaccines meet strict standards. Some governments even enforce mandatory vaccinations or restrict people's rights to opt out. The government cannot force a person to get a vaccination. However, it can impose penalties on people who choose not to participate in vaccination programs.

> "Today, with confidence in science & at the direction of the Office of the Attending Physician, I received the COVID-19 vaccine. As the vaccine is being distributed, we must all continue mask wearing, social distancing & other science-based steps to save lives & crush the virus."
>
> Nancy Pelosi, Speaker of the U.S. House of Representatives, in a tweet on December 18, 2020

◀ On November 9, 2020, during the COVID-19 pandemic, U.S. President-elect Joe Biden spoke about pharmaceutical company Pfizer's announcement that the vaccine it was testing was up to 90 percent effective in preventing the disease symptoms. The monitor here was in the briefing room of the White House in Washington, D.C.

NGO INVOLVEMENTS

A nongovernmental organization, or NGO, is any nonprofit unit that works independently of governments. Typically, NGOs support political or social causes, such as funding research and resources for global health concerns such as pandemics. They may work with governments, education institutes, global experts, research centers, private companies, and other organizations. The WHO, for example, works with member countries to reach and maintain high immunization levels in at-risk regions. The WHO advises on vaccine policies, strategies, research, and development. They also help build awareness of vaccines, educate about their safety and benefits, and ensure coverage for people who might not otherwise have access to information.

NOTEWORTHY ACTIONS

Gavi, the Vaccine Alliance, was created in 2000 to improve access to new and underused vaccines for vulnerable children in the world's poorest countries. Since then, it has vaccinated about 822 million children, resulting in more than 14 million lives saved and $150 billion in economic benefits.

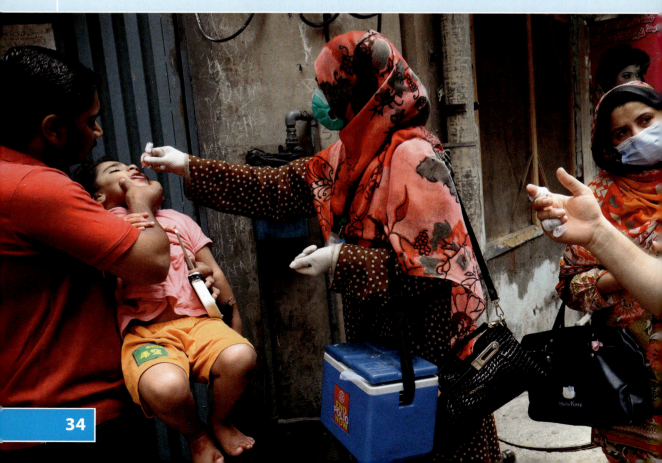

GLOBAL VACCINATION SUMMIT
BRUSSELS, 12 SEPTEMBER 2019

▲ The Global Vaccination Summit is a one-day event that brings together about 400 political, academic, health, and science leaders, as well as businesses, social media influencers, and NGOs. Its aim is to stimulate action against vaccine-preventable diseases and the spread of vaccine misinformation.

WHAT'S AT STAKE?

How has reading about different positions on vaccinations influenced or changed your understanding of the issue? What evidence do you think is the strongest? Why do you think this?

◄ During door-to-door polio vaccination campaigns in places such as Lahore, Pakistan, health care workers provide oral vaccines to help stop the spread of polio. Such campaigns were paused for several months during the COVID-19 pandemic, leading experts to fear polio cases will climb dramatically as a result. Polio is highly contagious and just one case can lead to many others.

A major funder of Gavi is the Bill & Melinda Gates Foundation. Each year, it also contributes to the cost of administering life-saving vaccines to people in need, as well as vaccine research and development, the latest science-and-technology innovations, and vaccine transportation. The foundation places a special focus on eradicating polio.

Since 1980, the United Nations Children's Fund (UNICEF) has played an important role in quadrupling global immunization rates. As a result, more than five lives are spared every minute. UNICEF's mission is to improve worldwide vaccination rates and stop disease in its tracks.

In many cases, there is a long delay between when a vaccine is developed and when it becomes available in the developing world. Johns Hopkins Bloomberg School of Public Health formed the International Vaccine Access Center (IVAC) that helps speed up access to vaccines by providing key decision makers with evidence-based vaccine information. IVAC also provides support to policymakers to help ensure better vaccine access, coverage, use, and funding.

5 THE CURRENT SITUATION

Once you get informed about a topic, it is important to stay up to date on the latest details. With vaccinations, the new disease COVID-19, which appeared in late 2019, is hot news. Vaccines for it are now being developed and tested. Facts and information about COVID-19 will change on a monthly basis.

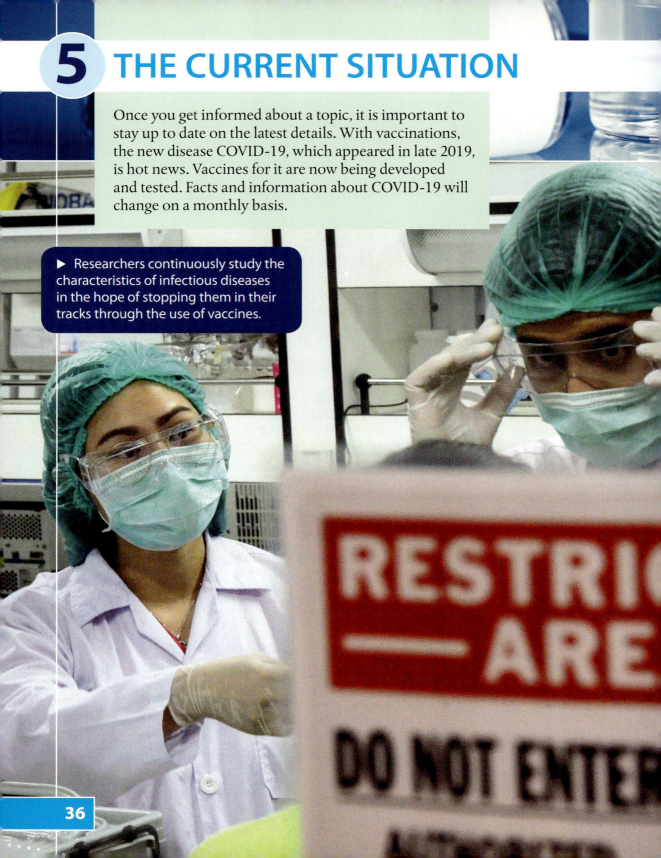

▶ Researchers continuously study the characteristics of infectious diseases in the hope of stopping them in their tracks through the use of vaccines.

KEY PLAYERS

The **Strategic Advisory Group of Experts on Immunization (SAGE)** is an advisory group that was founded by the WHO in 1999. It advises the WHO on global policies and strategies related to vaccines, including technology, research and development, administration, delivery, and more. SAGE advises on all types of vaccine-preventable diseases.

THE CENTRAL ISSUES

Why is it important for adults to update their vaccines? What can be done to create more awareness of adult vaccinations and stimulate more people to take action?

KEEPING TRACK

When new diseases are discovered, there is an urgent need to learn as much about them as quickly as possible. What pathogen is responsible? How is it caught and spread? Who is most vulnerable to it? Can a vaccine be developed to combat the disease? What can be done while a vaccine is being developed?

The WHO maintains a list of diseases for which vaccines are currently available. Its Vaccine Pipeline Tracker provides insight into the status of vaccine development around the world. For instance, researchers are working on a universal flu vaccine that will provide protection for several years rather than an annual injection. Other vaccines being tested include those against HIV and malaria.

ADULT VACCINATION

While most vaccines are given during childhood some, such as the vaccine for shingles, are given only to adults. The pneumococcal vaccine is mainly for at-risk individuals over a certain senior age. On top of that, many vaccines require boosters throughout life to maintain immunity.

Adults who were not vaccinated as children pose a risk of becoming infected with vaccine-preventable diseases and thereby infecting others and suffering the symptoms. Those adults may have been born in another country that did not offer certain vaccines, or perhaps new vaccines have become available since they were in school. As a result, herd immunity for some diseases is hard to achieve and some vaccines are underused.

VACCINE COVERAGE

Vaccination strategies must be closely monitored and assessed to ensure widespread coverage and effectiveness. The WHO began the Expanded Programme on Immunization (EPI) in 1974 with the goal of vaccinating children across the world. Originally, EPI worked to protect against six diseases—tuberculosis (BCG vaccine), diphtheria, tetanus, pertussis (DTP vaccine), measles, and poliomyelitis. Over time, the program expanded to include other vaccines and global initiatives.

THE DECADE OF VACCINES

In 2010, the global health community announced the Decade of Vaccines. The idea was to provide universal vaccine access to all by 2020. The WHO established the Global Vaccine Action Plan (GVAP) in 2012 to support the Decade of Vaccines. Many gains have been made, including a large increase in the number of vaccinated children, billions of dollars in economic productivity, and the development of several new vaccines. Yet, there are still many challenges to achieving the vision.

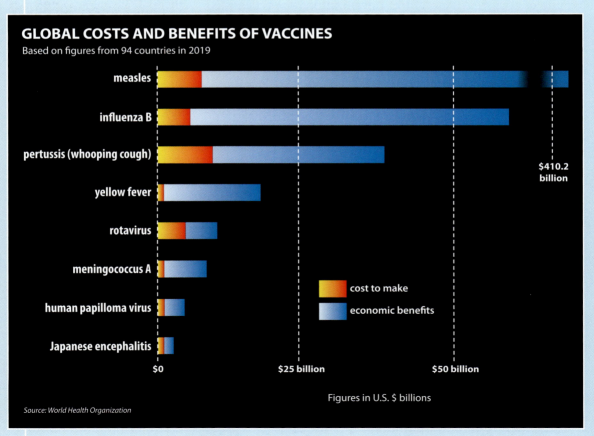

GLOBAL COSTS AND BENEFITS OF VACCINES
Based on figures from 94 countries in 2019

- measles — $410.2 billion
- influenza B
- pertussis (whooping cough)
- yellow fever
- rotavirus
- meningococcus A
- human papilloma virus
- Japanese encephalitis

cost to make
economic benefits

Figures in U.S. $ billions

Source: World Health Organization

Obstacles such as vaccine hesitancy, the capacity of health care workers and others needed to run vaccine programs, disease outbreaks, and poor supply chains, remain in the way.

RISING COSTS

There are many more trials and quality measures vaccine developers need to meet, and vaccine prices have risen over the years to cover the costs. There is a concern that the cost of vaccination programs is becoming too high to sustain them in developed and developing nations. As a result, some people and organizations are calling for vaccine costs to come down. However, others worry that lower prices would jeopardize research-and-development budgets and even cause some developers to stop making vaccines.

> "Helping young children live, get the right nutrition, contribute to their countries—that has a payback that goes beyond any typical financial return."
>
> Bill Gates, 2019, Microsoft co-founder and philanthropist, known for investing heavily in the fight against polio.

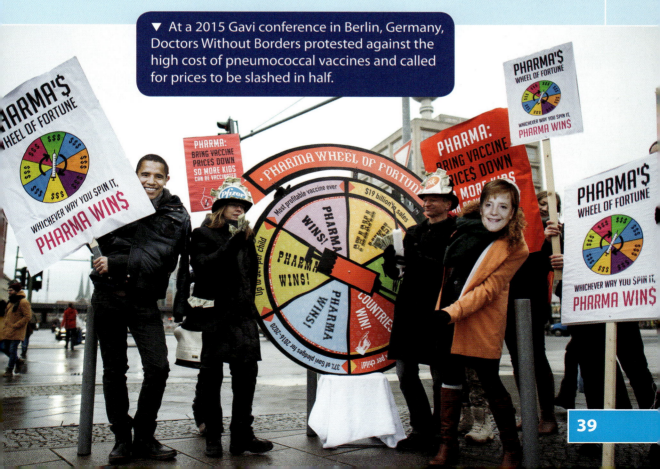

▼ At a 2015 Gavi conference in Berlin, Germany, Doctors Without Borders protested against the high cost of pneumococcal vaccines and called for prices to be slashed in half.

6 STAYING INFORMED

At times you may feel bombarded with information on current affairs—from classroom lessons, TV documentaries, Twitter feeds, radio programs, podcasts, newspaper headlines, let alone streaming data on the Internet. Vaccinations are also a very hot topic just now. But equipped with information literacy, you can get informed about it easily and stay informed by selecting good source materials.

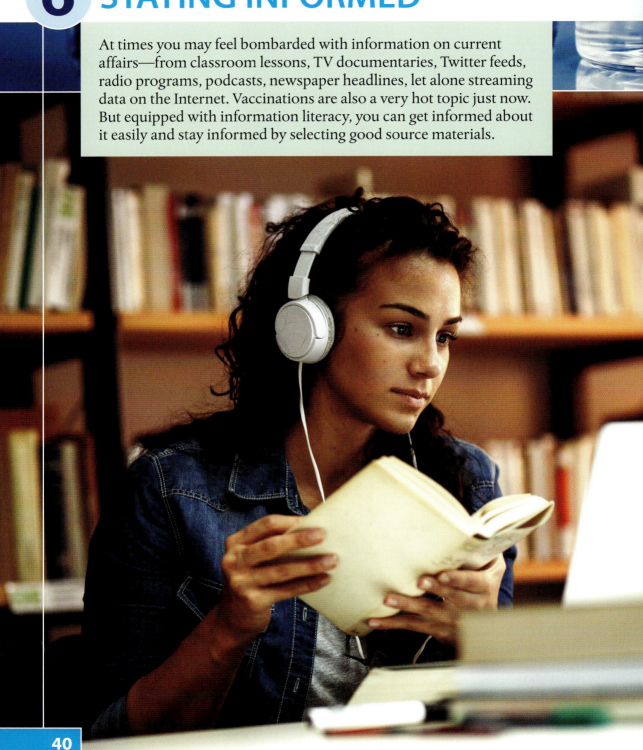

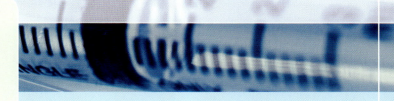

SEARCH TIPS
When looking at websites, address extensions can help pinpoint what sort of information you may be getting.

.gov (government): Restricted to use by government entities.

.org (organization): Anyone can register for this, although it is often used by nonprofit organizations and charities.

.com (commercial): Originally for businesses, this is the most widely used extension.

Country extensions:
- **.ca**   Canada
- **.au**   Australia
- **.uk**   United Kingdom
- **.ru**   Russia
- **.de**   Germany

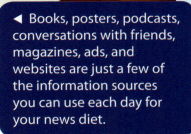

◀ Books, posters, podcasts, conversations with friends, magazines, ads, and websites are just a few of the information sources you can use each day for your news diet.

CREATE A NEWS DIET
By creating a balanced **news diet**, you'll get a healthy dose of daily updates from a variety of sources and perspectives in just a few minutes. A way to start is use Google Alerts on the Internet to monitor the web for content related to key search terms such as "vaccine development" or "immunization programs."

You can also look at news reports on diseases and vaccinations on websites for the WHO, the U.S. FDA, Health Canada, and Public Health Europe. For scientific studies, read articles in magazines such as *Scientific American*, *New Scientist*, and *Discover*. Tune into fact-based TV programs on CNN, *PBS NewsHour*, *CTV National News*, and NBC. Read articles in credible newspapers and magazines such as *The New York Times*, the *National Post*, *Time*, *Maclean's*, and *The Guardian*.

MEDIA LITERACY
"Fake news" refers to information that contains lies, bias, myths, and opinions. It is particularly common on social media. Media literacy is about using critical thinking skills to evaluate the source and the information presented. Is the information meant to entertain? Is anyone else reporting the same details? Are you getting the whole picture? Does the headline use sensationalism to grab your attention? Then it might be too good to be true. Don't take information at face value. On the Internet, Wikipedia keeps a list of fake news websites, and Snopes can help to debunk myths.

THE FUTURE OF VACCINE DEVELOPMENT

Currently, there are hundreds of new vaccines in the works. If successful, the vast majority—more than 130—will help prevent infectious diseases such as HIV, COVID-19, and malaria. Others hope to offer new treatment options or provide protection against cancers, autoimmune diseases, allergies, and other medical conditions, such as diabetes and Altzheimer's disease.

Research into vaccines has been a focus of science and technology for more than 40 years. The build up of knowledge means new vaccines can now be made in months not years, they are more effective than before, and they can provide stronger immunity. New vaccines may need fewer doses, too. All these innovations are very important when dealing with new threats and mutating viruses such as COVID-19 and influenza. The long and intense scientific research of vaccines also forms the main evidence to use against the views of anti-vaxxers.

NEW WAYS OF VACCINATION

Scientists are also discovering new ways to deliver vaccines without the use of injections that require trained health care professionals to administer. Vaccine patches, vaccine inhalers, and edible, plant-based vaccines are a few options being investigated. Such vaccines could also help improve supply chain and transportation issues, especially in developing countries and remote locations, since they are cheap to make and don't require cold storage.

Vaccination is one of the most cost-effective and successful medical interventions of the past two centuries. Most children today receive life-saving vaccines, with about one billion being immunized over the past decade alone. As a result of worldwide campaigns to vaccinate children, serious illness and deaths due to potentially deadly infectious diseases has decreased significantly. Smallpox has been eradicated, and polio cases have been reduced by 99 percent. Children everywhere have a better chance at reaching their full potential and lifespan as a result.

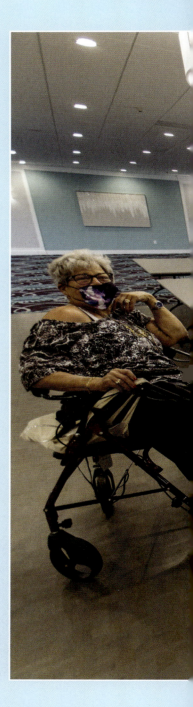

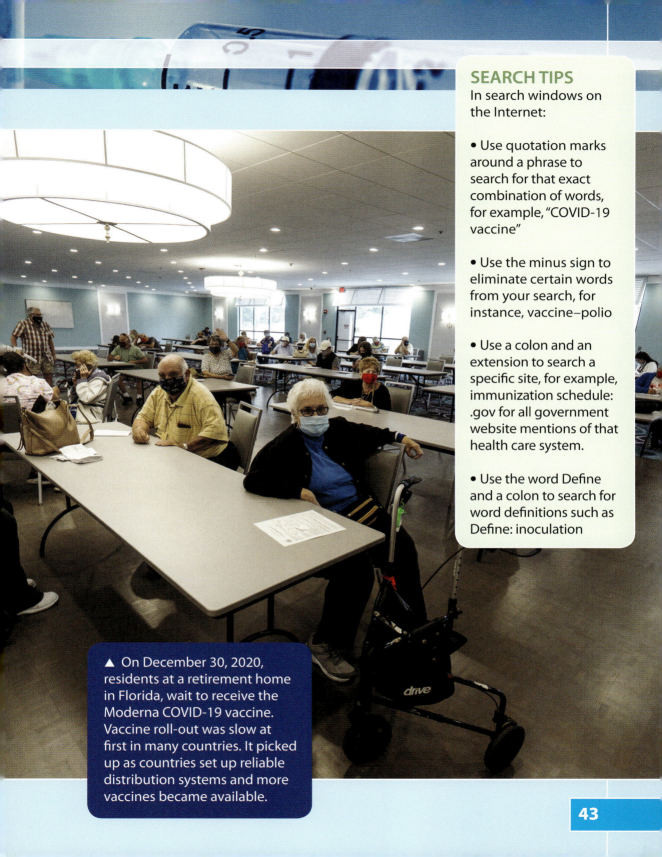

SEARCH TIPS
In search windows on the Internet:

• Use quotation marks around a phrase to search for that exact combination of words, for example, "COVID-19 vaccine"

• Use the minus sign to eliminate certain words from your search, for instance, vaccine–polio

• Use a colon and an extension to search a specific site, for example, immunization schedule: .gov for all government website mentions of that health care system.

• Use the word Define and a colon to search for word definitions such as Define: inoculation

▲ On December 30, 2020, residents at a retirement home in Florida, wait to receive the Moderna COVID-19 vaccine. Vaccine roll-out was slow at first in many countries. It picked up as countries set up reliable distribution systems and more vaccines became available.

GLOSSARY

administers Applies or dispenses

allergic reaction A response of the body's immune system to something it senses as harmful. It can cause swelling, difficulty breathing, and sometimes death

analyzing Studying carefully

antibodies Proteins produced by the immune system to fight off antigens

antigens Substances the immune system does not recognize and fights against

attenuated Reduced or weakened in effect, force, or value

bias Strong feelings for or against something

boosters Doses of a vaccine administered after the first one to raise the effectiveness of the vaccine

chronic Taking place over a long time or recurring, as with symptoms of some diseases

contagious Spread from one person or organism to another through direct or indirect contact

credible Trusted, reliable

current events Events happening now

economy How money is made, distributed, and spent in a certain country or region

efficacy The ability to achieve the desired outcome; effectiveness

epidemic A disease that spreads quickly to a large amount of people over a wide area

feces Waste material released from the bowels after food has been digested

genetic material The material that stores the genetic code of a plant, animal, or other organism; also known as DNA or RNA

herd immunity A population's ability to prevent the spread of a disease because the majority of people have been vaccinated or previously infected

historical societies Professional bodies preserving, collecting, and interpreting historical information

human right A basic right based on shared values that is believed to belong to every person in the world

immunity The body's ability to resist a disease

immunization The act of making someone immune to something, often through vaccination

maimed Scarred, disfigured, or permanently damaged

44

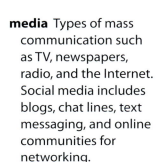

media Types of mass communication such as TV, newspapers, radio, and the Internet. Social media includes blogs, chat lines, text messaging, and online communities for networking.

microbiologist A scientist who studies microorganisms

news diet The sources you use to get your news

noncompliance Failing or refusing to comply with a rule or law

nongovernmental organizations (NGOs) Not-for-profit groups formed on a local, national, or international level that are not run by the government

outbreaks Sudden increases in cases of a disease

pandemic The spread of a new disease around the world

pathogen An organism that causes a disease; often called a germ

perspective Viewpoint

pharmaceutical Anything related to the manufacture, sale, and use of prescription drugs and vaccines

policies Ideas, plans, and procedures used to guide decision making

prevalence The proportion of people who have the same condition during a certain period of time

regulates Controls by a rule, standard, or law

sensationalist Intended to shock or excite

source materials Original documents or other pieces of evidence or key information

statistics A type of math that deals with the collection, analysis, and presentation of numerical data

stereotypes Widely held, but unfair and untrue, ideas or beliefs about what a person or group of people will be like

strain One of many forms of a bacterium or virus

supreme being God or other beings believed to have power over all things

synthesize To combine parts of different things

synthetic Made by a chemical process to imitate a natural substance

underserved Areas or people who are disadvantaged because they do not have access to suitable services

United Nations (UN) An organization of more than 170 countries and territories that formed in 1945 to help maintain peace and security around the world

SOURCE NOTES

QUOTATIONS
p. 4 https://tinyurl.com/y2enelr3
p. 6 https://tinyurl.com/y4qklqx7
p. 10 https://tinyurl.com/yxv2ygnv
p. 23 https://tinyurl.com/yy8gedc8
p. 29 https://tinyurl.com/y2ovlaa6
p. 33 https://tinyurl.com/y72ycvob
p. 39 https://tinyurl.com/y8t2kfrs

REFERENCES USED FOR THIS BOOK

Chapter 1: A Controversial Issue, pages 4–7
https://tinyurl.com/y255clsx
https://tinyurl.com/y3cg5pet
https://tinyurl.com/v58tcmb
https://tinyurl.com/yxcpzucg

Chapter 2: How to Get Informed, pages 8–13
https://tinyurl.com/y2wq2afh
https://tinyurl.com/y6ff225o
https://tinyurl.com/yxw6xfb9
https://tinyurl.com/y2jkyllk
https://tinyurl.com/yb39983g

Chapter 3: The Big Picture, pages 14–23
https://tinyurl.com/yy4kmrr3
https://tinyurl.com/y9nnmf2h
https://tinyurl.com/y7c72jwx
https://tinyurl.com/y4cfrd2v
https://tinyurl.com/yyk7n6ww
https://tinyurl.com/ybv28lew
https://tinyurl.com/y25p4rzn
https://tinyurl.com/yy5l9k88
https://tinyurl.com/y42xwux4
https://tinyurl.com/y5kyg4vr
https://tinyurl.com/jnq5anb
https://tinyurl.com/y5qb9xmv

Chapter 4: Making an Informed Decision, pages 24–35
https://tinyurl.com/y8hpavvy
https://tinyurl.com/yxr4hmet
https://tinyurl.com/tnk757r
https://tinyurl.com/y5x82fse
https://tinyurl.com/y4pxptlt
https://tinyurl.com/y5h3m4lx
https://tinyurl.com/yyoy9e5z
https://tinyurl.com/y4unh4o2
https://tinyurl.com/y67vjnzw
https://tinyurl.com/y8wvmgkq
https://tinyurl.com/y625k6bv

Chapter 5: The Current Situation, pages 36–39
https://tinyurl.com/yxud52gf
https://tinyurl.com/y7jgpj29
https://tinyurl.com/y462o3zf
https://tinyurl.com/yxtsb99r

Chapter 6: Staying Informed, pages 40–43
https://tinyurl.com/y4c3m6g9
https://tinyurl.com/y9ena64r
https://tinyurl.com/y4splxm4
https://tinyurl.com/yyx7tu8t
https://tinyurl.com/y3p36u2w

FIND OUT MORE

Finding good source material on the Internet can sometimes be a challenge. When analyzing how reliable the information is, consider these points:

- Who is the author of the page? Is it an expert in the field, or a person who experienced the event?

- Is the site well known and up to date? A page that has not been updated for several years probably has out-of-date information.

- Can you verify the facts with another site? Always double-check information.

- Have you checked all possible sites? Don't just look on the first page a search engine provides.

- Remember to try government sites and research papers.

- Have you recorded website addresses and names? Keep this data for a later time so you can backtrack and verify the information you want to use.

WEBSITES

Learn about the status of COVID-19 cases by country from Johns Hopkins University:
https://tinyurl.com/tztt3rn

Find out about vaccine safety:
www.vaccinesafetynet.org

Get information about European vaccinations:
https://vaccination-info.eu/en

Discover the facts about immunization in Canada:
https://immunize.ca

Learn more about the Centers for Disease Control and Prevention (CDC):
www.cdc.gov

Find out all about the WHO:
www.who.int

BOOKS

Jarrow, Gail. *Bubonic Panic: When Plague Invaded America*. Boyds Mills Press, 2016.

Koch, Falynn. *Plagues: The Microscopic Battlefield*. First Second, 2017.

Marrin, Albert. *Very, Very, Very Dreadful: The Influenza Pandemic of 1918*. Alfred A. Knopf, 2018.

Murphy, Jim, and Alison Blank. *Invincible Microbe: Tuberculosis and the Never-Ending Search for a Cure*. Houghton Mifflin Harcourt, 2015.

Peters, Marilee. *Patient Zero: Solving the Mysteries of Deadly Epidemics*. Annick Press, 2014.

Rooney, Anne, and David Antram. *You Wouldn't Want to Live Without Vaccinations!* Franklin Watts, 2015.

Squire, Ann O. *Flu*. Children's Press, 2017.

ABOUT THE AUTHOR

Heather C. Hudak has written hundreds of children's books on all types of topics. When she is not writing, Heather enjoys traveling all over the world. She also enjoys camping in the mountains near her home with her husband and their many rescue dogs and cats.

INDEX

allergic reaction 23
anthrax 7, 17
antibodies 5, 9, 18
antigens 18, 19
anti-vaccination, anti-vaxxers 11, 16, 17, 24, 27, 28–29, 31, 42

bias 7, 13, 41
boosters 23, 37, 42

children 5, 6, 7, 13, 15, 17, 19, 22, 25, 26, 27, 28, 29, 31, 32, 34, 37, 38, 39, 42
contagious diseases 6, 27, 35
COVID-19 26, 27, 29, 33, 35, 36, 42, 43
credibility 9, 12, 15, 25, 41

disease prevention 5, 6, 7, 9, 10, 15, 21, 23, 26, 27, 32, 33, 35, 37, 42, 43
diseases 4, 5, 6, 7, 9, 14, 15, 16, 19, 22, 23, 26, 28, 31, 32, 37, 41
doses 9, 20, 22, 23, 32, 41, 42

epidemic 14, 15

fake, false information 12, 27, 28, 35, 41
Food and Drug Administration (FDA), U.S. 21, 41

health care, services, systems 5, 6, 7, 10, 11, 15, 22, 26, 28, 30–31, 32, 41

hepatitis 7, 22
herd immunity 5, 9, 30, 31, 37
hesitancy 28–29, 30, 39

immune, immunity 5, 9, 16, 18, 19, 20, 21, 23, 28, 37, 42
immune system 18, 19, 27
immunization 9, 19, 34, 37, 38, 41, 42
influenza (flu) 21, 22, 37, 42
injections 9, 19, 21, 23, 42
inoculations 9, 21
Internet 9, 12, 40, 43

literacy skills 25, 40–41

measles 5, 7, 19, 23, 25, 28, 38
mumps 7, 19, 23, 28
myths 7, 13, 25, 30, 41

nongovernmental organizations (NGOs) 9, 34–35

oral doses 9, 23, 35
outbreaks 6, 14, 15, 27

pandemic 14, 15, 33, 34
pathogen 16, 18, 19, 20, 37
polio 5, 6, 17, 23, 32, 35, 38, 39, 42

rabies 7, 17
religious beliefs, views 5, 15, 24, 28
risks 7, 25, 27, 28, 32
rubella 7, 19, 22, 28

safety 5, 10, 12, 15, 21, 23, 24, 27, 29, 30, 34
science, vaccine 7, 9, 10, 11, 15, 29, 33, 35, 42
scientists 6, 9, 12, 13, 14, 15, 20, 21
side effects 16, 23, 27
smallpox 7, 16, 43
source material 11, 12–13, 25, 40–41
statistics 11
storage, vaccine 7, 19, 42

tetanus 7, 22, 26
toxins 19, 20
trials, vaccine 20–21
tuberculosis 7, 38

vaccination card, record 11
vaccination programs 4, 5, 7, 10, 11, 15, 22–23, 24, 25, 26–27, 29, 30, 31, 36, 39
vaccines 4, 5, 6, 9, 12, 13, 15, 16, 17, 18–19, 20–21, 22–23, 26, 27, 28, 30, 32, 33, 37, 38–39, 41, 42, 43
viewpoints 5, 12, 24, 41
viruses 15, 16, 17, 19, 23, 26, 27, 28, 33, 38, 42

whooping cough (pertussis) 7, 22, 23, 38
World Health Organization (WHO) 7, 9, 10, 16, 19, 34, 37, 38, 41

yellow fever 4, 11, 23, 38